Apple Cider Vinegar and Coconut Oil

Superfoods to Lose Weight, Look Younger and Improve Your Heath

Amanda Hopkins

Disclaimer: Every effort has been made to ensure the accuracy of the information contained in this book at the time of publication. The advice contained herein may not be suitable for your situation. The author and publisher do not assume any legal liability or responsibility for any loss or damage that may result from the use of the information in this book.

The contents in this book are for information and educational purposes only. The opinions and suggestions in this book are not intended to replace professional advice. If you have concerns about your health, please consult a doctor. It is always a good idea to consult a doctor before you use any natural remedy.

Sign Up for Free eBooks Newsletter

Thank you for downloading my book! At Insight Health Communications, we launch our ebooks for free for the first few days. By being a member of our free ebooks newsletter, you will be the first to know when new books launch so that you can download free books. We won't send you any spam and you can opt-out at any time. Click the link below to access the newsletter now and thanks again for your support!

http://www.insightweightloss.com/freebooksignuppage.html

Table of Contents

Chapter 1: Introduction to Apple Cider Vinegar

If you don't already have apple cider vinegar handy in your pantry, it's a good idea to get some. This natural remedy can take care of your minor ailments, such as hiccups, and it can also tackle chronic issues such as diabetes and heart disease. It's being used for weight loss and common colds. This introduction of apple cider vinegar will give you a glimpse of what it is and what it can do.

Apple Cider Vinegar: What Is It?

There are lots of different vinegars on the market, and they have all been used for things like cleaning and cooking. If you color Easter eggs every year, you probably use vinegar to create the egg dye. Apple cider vinegar is becoming a very popular form of vinegar, especially among people who believe in natural health and holistic medicine. It's fermented crushed apples and it looks a little bit like a glass of cider or apple juice. It's low in calories, with only a few calories per tablespoon. It tastes sweet and acidic and you might have a hard time drinking it straight from the bottle.

Apple Cider Vinegar's Active Ingredients

Apple cider vinegar contains apples and yeast. When those two components are combined, the sugars begin to ferment and turn into alcohol. Bacteria are added to the mixture, creating acetic acid. That acid has the ability to kill many different types of bacteria. You can use it to clean and disinfect household appliances and it also takes care of warts, lice, ear infections and fungus. The acetic acid in this vinegar can preserve food and protect it against dangerous bacteria such as E. coli. In addition to killing bacteria, the acid in apple cider vinegar can prevent existing bacteria from growing or multiplying, giving you a chance to heal and surfaces a chance to stay clean.

Chlorogenic acid is also present in apple cider vinegar, and that can battle heart disease, particularly by attacking bad cholesterol levels in your blood. Studies are being conducted to see what kind of effects it has on blood pressure and weight loss. Many types of vinegar are known to regulate blood sugar and help with the processing of insulin, which is why apple cider vinegar is used to help people suffering from diabetes.

Choosing an Apple Cider Vinegar

Consuming apple cider vinegar has no known side effects and it won't damage your health. There are many different types of vinegars that can be purchased in stores and online. Many natural health experts recommend you look for a brand that includes the "mother." The mother is found in organic, unfiltered apple cider vinegar. It preserves the strands of protein, enzymes and healthy bacteria. You'll know your vinegar contains the mother when it looks a bit cloudy and seems to have a web-like appearance.

The alternative is sparkling vinegar or a refined, clear product that you can find commercially. While this type of apple cider vinegar may also have brilliant benefits for you health, it's not as packed with protein and enzymes as the organic varieties. The processed vinegar could strip out some of the best health advantages. Even though the vinegars with the "mother" might look off-putting, ugly apple cider vinegars are often the best to use.

This introduction of apple cider vinegar is meant to help you understand what it is and how it can help you. Whether you want to lose weight, control your diabetes or protect yourself against infections, bacteria and even some forms of cancer, this product can help you feel better. It's natural and safe, so you have nothing to lose by incorporating it into your life.

Chapter 2: Exploring the Health Benefits of Apple Cider Vinegar

The health benefits of apple cider vinegar extend to preventing the growth of cancer cells, managing diabetes and protecting your heart from cardiovascular issues. It can also be helpful with minor health issues and used for general day to day upkeep. If you're looking for a natural and easy remedy to one of these common conditions, try some apple cider vinegar.

Apple Cider Vinegar for Weight Loss

If you're someone who has struggled with weight for a large part of your life, or even if there's just a stubborn five pounds that you cannot seem to drop; apple cider vinegar can help you lose and maintain weight. It has a stabilizing effect on your blood sugar and it helps you metabolize fats and nutrients a lot better.

The Journal of Functional Foods recently published a study that showed drinking apple cider vinegar before meals can lower your blood sugar. It's a simple recipe: mix one tablespoon of apple cider vinegar into an 8 ounce glass of water and drink it. That will bring your body's glucose level down. It will block the starch you eat and keep it from being converted into fat. That will help you drop unwanted pounds and give you a better shot at maintaining a healthy weight.

Apple Cider Vinegar for Skin Care

If you're using a lot of heavily scented, expensive beauty products and you're not thrilled with the results - try something different. Apple cider vinegar has a lot to offer your skin and it works especially well as a facial wash. It can also help to treat age spots and unsightly pimples and acne. This natural product is safer for you, and you have a better chance of leaving your skin feeling new and refreshed.

Make your own facial cleanser by diluting a little apple cider vinegar. Don't put it directly on your skin because it's very strong and can do damage on its own. Mix two tablespoons of vinegar with two tablespoons of water. Add a tablespoon of green tea. Apply the mixture to your face with a cotton ball. Keep it away from your eyes and if you're using this cleanser to treat acne, you might feel a slight stinging sensation on those pimples. You'll easily and safely remove makeup, dirt and oil.

Apple Cider Vinegar for Foot Fungus

One of the most common types of fungus occurs on the feet. Toenails are especially susceptible and it can be disturbing for people who suffer from it. The fungus creates an unsightly, yellow and brittle toenail. Before too long, the nail starts to crumble and it can be very painful. Apple cider vinegar can fight off the fungus and keep it from spreading to other parts of your foot. It's a safe natural remedy that's easy to create and the anti-viral and anti-bacterial properties in the vinegar will have an immediate and lasting effect.

Add two cups of apple cider vinegar to two cups of water in a bowl. Soak the affected foot for 15 minutes. Add two tablespoons of baking soda to the solution and stir. Put your foot back in the mixture for another 15 minutes. Pat your foot dry. Do this every day for at least a week and you'll notice a dramatic improvement in your foot fungus.

Apple Cider Vinegar for Yeast Infections

Yeast and bacteria is present in the body, and in many cases it serves a positive purpose. When too much bad yeast and bacteria take over the bodily systems, however, uncomfortable conditions can be the result.

Yeast that grows out of control in the gut is called Candida, and apple cider vinegar can be useful in fighting off this type of infection. Chronic vaginal yeast infections can also benefit from natural remedies including apple cider vinegar.

Using antibiotics puts you at risk for making the infection worse. Instead, deal with yeast problems naturally. Drink an 8 ounce glass of water with a tablespoon of apple cider vinegar. Drink it on an empty stomach when possible. Drink this twice a day to treat your yeast infection. Take a bath and add 2 cups of vinegar to your water. This will also help relieve your symptoms. Soak for at least 15 minutes and then dry yourself thoroughly.

Apple Cider Vinegar to Prevent Flu

The flu inspires dread and fear throughout all populations of people. Its symptoms include fever, chills and aches, coughing, sore throat and a generally weakened body. While the flu vaccine seems like it should prevent the illness from getting to you, lots of people still manage to get the flu even after being vaccinated. There are so many different strains of the flu virus that the medical establishment can hardly keep up.

Apple cider vinegar is an effective treatment for your flu symptoms. It can help minimize your cough, soothe your sore throat and provide some relief for sinus problems that are often associated with compromised immune systems and colds and flu viruses. When you have the flu, your body becomes more acidic in general. The apple cider vinegar has an alkaline effect when it's doing battle against the flu virus, bringing you relief and minimizing what could be a long lasting illness.

Make yourself a tea that will feel good on your throat and give your body the necessary ingredients to fight the flu. Mix 2 tablespoons of apple cider vinegar to 8 ounces of hot water. Add 2 tablespoons of honey and stir. Drink the tea at least twice a day while you are recovering from the flu and if you feel like you're getting sick, cut off the symptoms by drinking the tea as often as possible.

The health benefits of apple cider vinegar are unique. The acidic components of the vinegar provide a number of antibacterial properties and it also beats back the viruses that threaten to disrupt the ecosystem of your body. Use it when you can as your go-to home remedy and you'll find your weight, skin, nails and overall health will begin to improve and feel right again.

Chapter 3: Enjoying Apple Cider Vinegar Recipes

Understanding the fantastic health benefits of this potent vinegar should have you stockpiling apple cider vinegar recipes. You can incorporate this natural remedy into quite a few of your foods and you'll find yourself feeling better, looking better and taking better care of yourself. Whether you want to lose weight, fight off infections or protect yourself from viruses, apple cider vinegar can help you boost your immunity and lead a more holistic life.

Apple Cider Dressing

If you don't like drinking apple cider in water or tea, try it on your vegetables with this simple dressing.

Ingredients:

1/4 cup apple cider vinegar

1/4 cup white wine vinegar

1 tablespoon spicy mustard

1/3 cup olive oil

1 clove of garlic, minced

2 shallots, minced

Directions:

Whisk everything together in a small bowl and drizzle over your favorite salad. This recipe makes about a cup of salad dressing and covers at least two salads.

Lemon Pepper Salad Dressing

Salads are excellent for weight loss and good health. Dress your next one with a little apple cider vinegar, and you'll never use a bottled brand again.

Ingredients:

1/2 cup apple cider vinegar

1/2 cup extra virgin olive oil

1 teaspoon red pepper flakes

1 teaspoon black pepper

1 teaspoon white pepper

1 teaspoon sea salt

2 lemons, juiced

Directions:

Whisk together the vinegar, peppers, lemon juice and salt. Slowly pour in the olive oil until it's completely incorporated.

Pour into a jar or bottle that can be sealed and refrigerate for at least 30 minutes.

This recipe makes one cup of salad dressing and can serve two people.

Honey Cider Vinaigrette

It tastes great as a salad dressing and this vinaigrette also works well as a marinade when you're roasting, baking or grilling your favorite protein.

Ingredients:

1/4 cup apple cider vinegar

3/4 cup extra virgin olive oil

2 tablespoons honey

3 tablespoons water

1 tablespoon dried rosemary

1 tablespoon dried thyme

Salt and pepper

Directions:

Combine all ingredients in a jar with a lid and shake hard until everything is combined. Add extra salt and pepper or dried herbs for taste as necessary.

This recipe makes about one cup of vinaigrette and serves as dressing for two salads or makes a nice marinade for two servings of chicken, meat or fish.

Spicy Ketchup

If you're looking for an adventurous condiment, this is the one.

Ingredients:

3 tablespoons apple cider vinegar

6 tomatoes, chopped

3 celery stalks

1 yellow onion, diced

2 tablespoons dark brown sugar

1 tablespoon red pepper flakes

1 teaspoon chili powder

1/4 cup water

1 teaspoon salt

1 teaspoon pepper

Directions:

Put water in a saucepan and boil the onion and celery for 20 minutes.

In another pan, cook the tomatoes, salt and pepper for 30 minutes until they are soft and turning to liquid. Add the onions and celery.

Put everything, including the spices, into a blender and pulse until all the vegetables are liquid and combined.

Allow it to cool and refrigerate. This recipe makes three cups of ketchup.

Cranberry Smoothie

The antioxidants in the cranberries will complement those in the vinegar. This is a frothy, frozen treat that can taste like more of a dessert than a smoothie.

Ingredients:

2 tablespoons apple cider vinegar

2 cups water

1/2 cup ice

1/2 cup frozen cranberries

2 teaspoons maple syrup

1 lime, juiced

Directions:

Combine all the ingredients in a blender. Blend until the ice and cranberries break down and everything is mixed. This recipe makes one smoothie.

Mango Fruit Smoothie

This smoothie is a great way to start your day if you don't feel like making a big breakfast.

Ingredients:

2 tablespoons apple cider vinegar

1/2 mango, peeled and chopped

1/2 banana

1/4 cup frozen blueberries

1/2 cup almond milk

Directions:

Combine everything in a blender and mix it on high. This recipe makes one smoothie.

Sausage and Apples

Sweet and tart, this recipe combines the healthier turkey sausage with an abundance of apples.

Ingredients:

1/4 cup apple cider vinegar

6 turkey sausages

2 cups white wine

2 apples, peeled and cored

1 tablespoon butter

1 tablespoon cinnamon

Directions:

In a large skillet, cook the sausages in the white wine over medium heat with a cover on the pan. Cook until the wine nearly evaporates, about 20 minutes.

Remove the sausages from the pan and add the chopped apples, the apple cider vinegar and the butter. Stir until the apples are coated in liquid and butter and cook for 10 minutes, until the apples get soft and begin to brown. Add the cinnamon to the pan and mix.

Top the sausage with the apple mixture. This recipe serves three people.

Chicken and Onions

This variation on a French recipe using red wine vinegar is healthy and low in calories, even with the little bit of butter.

Ingredients:

1 cup apple cider vinegar

4 chicken breasts

3 tablespoon olive oil

1 red onion, sliced

1 tablespoon butter

Salt and pepper

Directions:

Heat olive oil in a skillet over medium high heat. Season the chicken with salt and pepper and heat in the skillet for five minutes on each side, until brown.

Remove chicken and add onions to the pan, stirring and cooking for two minutes. Add the apple cider vinegar and raise the heat to high. Cook for five minutes, stirring.

Add the butter and allow the sauce to thicken. Return the chicken to the skillet and stir with the vinegar and onions for two minutes.

This recipe serves four people.

Rice and Beans

It's simple and economical; a pleasing plate of steaming rice and beans. When you cook it with apple cider vinegar, you also get the associated health benefits.

Ingredients:

1 tablespoon apple cider vinegar

1 cup brown rice

1 can black beans, rinsed

1/2 cup chopped onion

1/2 cup chopped green pepper

1 tablespoon olive oil

2 tomatoes, chopped

1 garlic clove, chopped

1 teaspoon thyme

2 teaspoons cayenne

1 teaspoon red pepper flakes

Directions:

Heat olive oil in a sauce pan and sauté onion, green pepper, garlic, tomatoes, thyme, cayenne and red pepper flakes. After five minutes, add the vinegar, rice and beans. Bring to a boil.

Lower heat and cook at a simmer for 20 minutes. This recipe makes 4 servings.

Potato Salad

For picnics or even as a main dish, this hearty potato salad relies on apple cider vinegar for its zesty dressing.

Ingredients:

3 tablespoons apple cider vinegar

1/4 cup olive oil

1 lemon, juiced

2 pounds red bliss potatoes

2 green onions, sliced

1 clove garlic, minced

1 teaspoon celery seeds

1 teaspoon paprika

2 tablespoons fresh dill

Salt and pepper to taste

Directions:

Boil whole potatoes until tender. Cool and cut into cubes. Toss with the green onions and garlic.

In a separate bowl, whisk the olive oil, vinegar, lemon juice, celery seed, paprika, dill, salt and pepper. Cover the potatoes and mix.

This recipe serves 5 or 6 people as a side dish.

These apple cider vinegar recipes are easy to make and tasty to enjoy. You can also try substituting apple cider vinegar for other vinegars that you come across in your favorite recipes. It will bring a fresher, fruit-filled flavor to your best loved foods, and you'll be doing your body a favor. Remember that in addition to adding this powerful ingredient to the food you cook, it does well as a drink or stirred into teas.

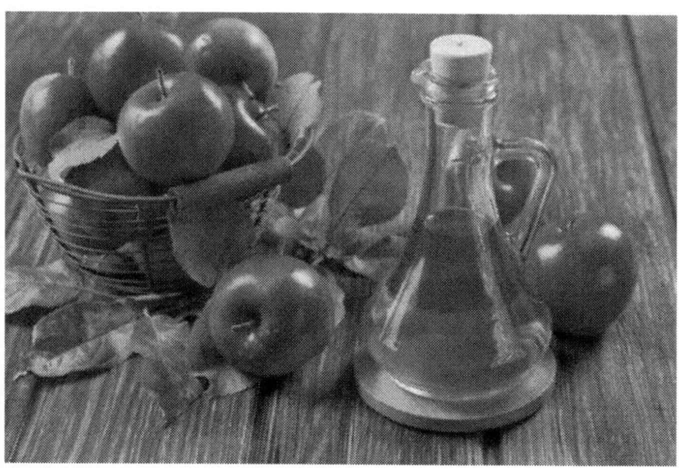

Chapter 4: An Introduction to Coconut Oil

Coconut oil is showing up in a lot of beauty products, health supplements and even recipes. This introduction of coconut oil is written for people who want to harness its power but may not understand exactly what it is and what it can do. Once you get to know the benefits and values of coconut oil, you'll want to incorporate it into several parts of your daily life.

Explaining Coconut Oil - What is It?

Coconut oil is extracted from mature coconuts. It's pressed from the coconut palm in either a dry pressing process or a wet process. This type of oil is safe to ingest and it contains a lot of fat. It's used in cooking, and many people have effectively lost weight and lowered their cholesterol levels by using coconut oil.

If you're less concerned with health and more concerned with taste, its sweet and nutty flavor also makes it an ideal oil to use for frying and baking. It also contains medicinal properties. People utilize coconut oil for help with heart disease, chronic fatigue illnesses, bowel irregularities, thyroid problems and help with their immune systems.

Coconut oil has also been useful as a skin moisturizer. It brings added protein to hair and nails and it is used in many soaps.

Active Components of Coconut Oil

The most active ingredients in coconut oil are the medium-chain triglycerides. While these are saturated fats, they are not as dangerous as some of the other types of fats that you want to avoid putting in your body. Trans fats, for example, can do far more damage than the type of fat found in coconut oil. Saturated fats that come from animal products are also worse for your health than the fat you get from coconut oil.

A large amount of lauric acid is present in coconut oil. This substance has been found to fight the bad cholesterol that can gather in your blood. There is also linoleic acid in coconut oil, which is a monounsaturated fatty acid. This acid promotes bone health, according to scientists at the University of Maryland Medical Center. It can also reduce problems with inflammation.

Choosing a Good Coconut Oil

There are a number of different kinds of coconut oil on the market. You'll see a huge range in prices and also labels like "cold pressed," "virgin" and "refined." Make sure you're choosing a high quality coconut oil that delivers on all its promises.

The first distinction is refined coconut oil and unrefined coconut oil. Refined oil has been processed, so it doesn't deliver all of the same health benefits as an unrefined oil, which is delivered to consumers in its raw form. Unrefined coconut oil might also be called virgin coconut oil or extra-virgin coconut oil. It simply means there have been no chemicals or additives included in it during the pressing process.

Extraction methods also differ. You can choose a cold-pressed coconut oil, an expeller-pressed oil or a centrifuged oil. Coconut oil can withstand high levels of heat, so the method of extraction doesn't always matter. There is less heat used in the centrifuged coconut oil, which contributes to a mild and less intense flavor.

With this introduction of coconut oil, you have hopefully learned what it can do for you and how to buy it. Read the bottles and the labels carefully so you know what kind of extraction method was used and whether it is refined. As you begin to use it more often in your cooking and personal habits, you'll grow more confident with your ability to pick out exactly what kind of coconut oil you need.

Chapter 5: Health Benefits of Coconut Oil

Coconut oil has a number of health benefits, and it can be used to solve health problems and protect you from toxins and environmental threats. In places where it is naturally found, such as tropical islands, local cultures use it extensively. It seems a new health benefit of coconut oil is being discovered on a regular basis. Years ago, there were concerns about the high levels of fat in coconut oil, but further research and study has demonstrated that the lauric acid present in coconut oil does a lot of good, and the saturated fat is quickly turned into energy and can boost metabolism.

Health Benefit of Coconut Oil

The lauric acid found in coconut oil allows the body to fight off viruses, bacteria and the diseases that can develop when the body is out of balance. It boosts your immune system and protects you against cardiovascular problems and illnesses as powerful as influenza. Recent studies suggest that coconut oil can help starve off cancer cells, reduce the symptoms and improve the quality of life of breast cancer patients.

The digestive system also benefits from coconut oil. If you suffer from irritable bowel syndrome or other forms of gastro-intestinal distress, the acids and fats in the coconut oil will bring you relief and protect your system from further damage. It also helps your body to absorb the nutrients and minerals it needs, including amino acids.

Applying coconut oil to infections can also have an immediate and soothing effect. Whether it's a cold sore, ringworm, an inflamed abrasion or even a bruise, a layer of coconut oil will protect the area from dust and toxins floating around in the air, allowing the tissue's healing process to begin and to act more effectively.

Skin Care Benefit of Coconut Oil

Massage oils and moisturizers often contain coconut oil and that's because it has the ability to soften and soothe your skin. It's safe to apply directly to the skin if you don't want to use products that have other ingredients added to them. You'll notice that dry or flaky skin responds well to the oil, and its solid nature will begin to melt on contact with your skin, and rub right into whatever affected areas need it.

If you're worried about the aging process, use this oil to delay the onset of wrinkles and sagging or pulling. It will keep your skin taut, shiny and youthful. There are a number of antioxidants in coconut oil that keep your skin nourished and healthy. Rub a pea-sized amount of coconut oil to the skin right underneath your eyes, and in the corners where you might see the early development of crow's feet. Doing this on a regular basis will beat back the wrinkles and keep your delicate skin smooth and protected.

Skin diseases and afflictions also respond well to this particular oil. It treats eczema, psoriasis and dermatitis. Remember that a little bit goes a long way; you don't want to lather yourself in coconut oil or you'll feel greasy and slippery. Simply apply a little bit to a small area on your skin, and you'll love the results.

Hair Care Benefit of Coconut Oil

Like skin, your hair needs protein and natural moisturizers in order to grow, stay healthy and look shiny. Coconut oil can be found in a number of shampoos, conditioners and other hair products. However, you can apply it directly to your hair and still get excellent results without including a lot of the chemicals and perfumes that are found in commercial products.

Combing coconut oil through your hair after every shampoo can help to repair damaged hair and generate new growth. It can work well on your scalp, too. Massaging this oil into your scalp can prevent dandruff, even if your scalp is always dry and itchy. Some people use it as a natural remedy to head lice. Not only can it kill the lice that might be in the hair already, it can also prevent the growth of any lice eggs.

Make yourself a nourishing hair mask by mixing together one tablespoon of coconut oil with one tablespoon of raw honey. Heat the mixture in a saucepan over low heat. Once it's combined and cooled, apply it to your hair, starting at the scalp and working your way down to the roots. Allow the hair mask to soak into your hair and leave it on for at least half an hour. Then, rinse it out in the shower and dry your hair. You'll find your hair is a lot softer, smoother and easier to manage.

Weight Loss Benefit of Coconut Oil

With its high fat content, you might be suspicious that coconut oil can really help you lose weight. However, it's very effective in regulating your metabolism and helping you shed unwanted pounds and extra fat. It's an easy oil to digest, which means your body won't store it as fat; instead, it will put the fatty acids and numerous nutrients to good use. The compounds in this oil have a positive effect on your thyroid and endocrine system, which are two things that play a major role in regulating your weight and keeping you from putting on extra pounds.

Eating a tablespoon of coconut oil before every meal will help maintain a healthy blood sugar and keep you from overeating. If melting the oil in your mouth and swallowing it seems distasteful, mix the coconut oil into a glass of water or your favorite tea. Drinking this mixture three times a day will help your body metabolize fat and keep you looking and feeling great.

These are just a few of the health benefits of coconut oil. If you train yourself to cook with it regularly and to use it as part of your beauty routine, you'll be able to lose weight, defy the aging process and keep your hair and skin smooth and shiny.

Chapter 6: Enjoying Coconut Oil Recipes

These coconut oil recipes can help you harness the power of this nutrition-packed ingredient. It's an excellent oil to cook with, and you'll find it adds flavor and ease to your cooking. Take advantage of the taste as well as the health benefits.

Cranberry Granola

Whether you like granola as a breakfast cereal or sprinkled on top of your fruit and yogurt, this recipe is nutty, fruity and delicious.

Ingredients:

1/4 cup coconut oil

3 cups old fashioned oats

1/2 cup dried cranberries

1/2 cup crushed walnuts

1/4 teaspoon cinnamon

1/2 cup water

1/4 cup butter

1/4 cup honey

1/4 cup whole cane sugar

Directions:

Preheat your oven to 350 degrees F. Melt the coconut oil in a saucepan over low heat and add honey, butter, sugar, water and cinnamon.

Spread the oats in a baking pan and then add the melted liquid mixture, stirring everything together. Bake for 20 minutes.

Remove the pan and stir. Bake for another 15 minutes. Allow the mixture to cool for 10 minutes and then add the cranberries and walnuts.

This recipe makes five servings that are one cup each.

Garlic Hummus Dipping Sauce

Perfect for a plate of raw veggies or some crispy crackers, this hummus uses coconut oil instead of olive oil.

Ingredients:

2 tablespoons melted coconut oil

3 cloves of garlic

1/4 cup plain yogurt

2 cups garbanzo beans

1/4 cup water

Salt and pepper

Directions:

In a mini chopper or blender, combine all the ingredients and pulse until they are chopped and combined.

Use a spatula or spoon to scrape the pulpy parts off the sides of the blender. Scoop everything out and into a dish, adding salt and pepper to taste.

This recipe makes about three cups of hummus, serving as a snack or appetizer for six to eight people.

Blueberry Banana Smoothie

For a refreshing snack or an energizing breakfast, this smoothie does the job. It includes coconut milk as well as coconut oil, giving you an extra blast of tropical flavor.

Ingredients:

1 tablespoon coconut oil

6 ounces coconut milk

1/2 cup blueberries

1/2 banana

2 tablespoons plain yogurt

8-10 ice cubes

Directions:

Put the ice cubes in a blender and then add the fruits, yogurt and coconut oil. Pour the coconut milk on top and blend until smooth. This recipe makes one smoothie.

Strawberry Vanilla Smoothie

The slow addition of melted coconut oil to this smoothie will give it a milder flavor, allowing you to savor the vanilla and strawberry tones instead. This recipe is full of antioxidants and strength for your immune system.

Ingredients:

2 tablespoons melted coconut oil

1/2 cup plain yogurt

1 teaspoon vanilla extract

1 cup almond milk

10 strawberries

1/2 cup ice

Directions:

Add everything except the coconut oil to the blender and mix. Slowly add the coconut oil while everything is being blended. This recipe makes one smoothie.

Italian Chicken Stir Fry

This recipe combines protein, veggies and a heart healthy dose of coconut oil. Serve it with a side salad or all by itself.

Ingredients:

2 tablespoons coconut oil

8 ounces chicken tenders, cut into one inch chunks

2 cups broccoli

2 cloves garlic, minced

1/2 cup red onion, sliced

1 cup grape tomatoes

2 cups kale

3 tablespoons red wine vinegar

Salt and pepper

Directions:

Cook the chicken in the coconut oil on a large skillet over medium heat. It should brown within 10 minutes.

Add the onion, garlic, broccoli, tomatoes and kale. Continue cooking for another five minutes, until kale has wilted and everything is combined.

Remove from heat and toss with red wine vinegar. Add salt and pepper to taste. This recipe serves two people.

Grilled Cheese

There's no comfort food like a grilled cheese. Substitute coconut oil for the unhealthy butter, and you have a better sandwich.

Ingredients:

2 slices whole grain bread

2 slices provolone cheese

1 slice cheddar cheese

2 slices tomato

1 tablespoon coconut oil, divided

Directions:

Layer the cheese slices and then the tomato on top of one piece of bread and cover it with the other piece of bread.

Heat a skillet or pan and melt half of the tablespoon of coconut oil in it. Spread the other half tablespoon of coconut oil on top of the sandwich.

Cook for three or four minutes on each side, until the bread is crispy and brown. This recipe makes one grilled cheese sandwich.

Lemon Lime Rice

The citrus smell and taste of this rice goes well with fish or chicken.

Ingredients:

2 tablespoons coconut oil

1 cup brown rice

1/4 cup coconut flakes

1 cup coconut milk

1 cup vegetable broth

1 lime, juiced

1 lemon, juiced

Directions:

Rinse rice and drain. Heat coconut oil in a large skillet. Add rice and coconut flakes and combine, stirring for five minutes.

Add lime juice and lemon juice, stir for one more minute. Add the milk and broth. Bring to a boil, then reduce heat to low. Cover the mixture and allow it to simmer for 20 minutes.

Remove from heat and keep it covered for an additional five minutes. This recipe makes four servings that are 1/2 cup each.

Spicy Corn on the Cob

Again, by eliminating butter and using coconut oil instead, you're getting a healthier dish and a fresher taste.

Ingredients:

4 ears of corn, shucked and rinsed

1/4 cup coconut oil

2 limes

2 teaspoons red pepper flakes

Directions:

Melt the coconut oil in a small saucepan. Boil the ears of corn and allow them to cool.

Add the juice of the limes to the melted oil and sprinkle in the red pepper flakes. With a sharp knife, cut the corn kernels off the cob and into a bowl.

Pour the oil mixture over the corn and toss. This recipe serves four.

Super Salad

Get as creative as you want with this recipe; add the salad ingredients you like most, and don't be afraid to include some protein, like tuna, hard boiled eggs or some chopped chicken.

Ingredients:

3 cups romaine lettuce

3 cups baby spinach

3 cups red leaf lettuce

1/2 cucumber, sliced

1/4 cup sundried tomatoes

1 carrot, chopped

1 celery stalk, chopped

1/4 cup pine nuts

2 tablespoons coconut oil, melted

1/2 lime, juiced

1 tablespoon apple cider vinegar

1 teaspoon black pepper

Directions:

Bring your salad veggies to room temperature. Combine the lettuces and vegetables in a large bowl.

Heat the coconut oil over low heat, adding the lime juice and vinegar. Pour it over the salad, mixing in the pine nuts. Sprinkle with pepper.

This recipe makes one entrée-size salad or two side salads.

Herb Infused Eggs

A hot breakfast that will give you fuel throughout the day, the coconut oil in this recipe is tasty as well as functional. It will keep your eggs from sticking to your pan.

Ingredients:

1 tablespoon coconut oil

4 large eggs

1/4 cup coconut milk

1 tablespoon dried basil

1 tablespoon dried sage

1 tablespoon dried cilantro

Salt and pepper

Directions:

Heat the coconut oil in a frying pan. Beat the eggs with the coconut milk until combined. Add the dried herbs.

Scramble eggs in the hot pan. Sprinkle with salt and pepper to taste. This recipe serves two.

These coconut oil recipes are healthy, tasty and easy to make. Give them a try and remember - you can always eat coconut oil right out of the jar. No recipe needed.

Conclusion

Apple cider vinegar and coconut oil are exceptional natural remedies and health supplements. I hope this book helps you incorporate these superfoods into your daily life to lose weight, look younger and improve your health.

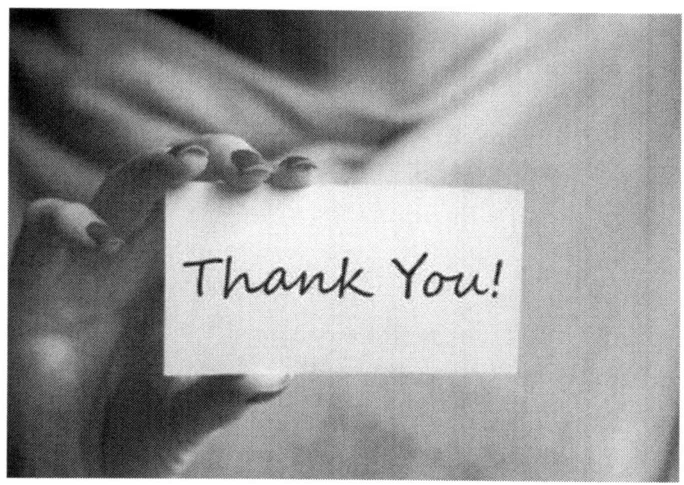

Finally, I want to thank you again for downloading this book. If you enjoyed the book, please take the time to share your thoughts and post a review on the Apple Cider Vinegar and Coconut Oil Amazon book page. It would be greatly appreciated!

For more information about free ebooks on healthy living and weight loss, please sign up for my free ebook newsletter at http://www.insightweightloss.com/freebooksignuppage.html.

Best wishes,

Amanda Hopkins

Preview of "Sugar Detox: Sugar Detox Recipes to Beat Sugar Addiction, Lose Weight and Achieve Optimal Health"

Chapter 1: Acknowledging the Addiction to Sugar

If you've never heard about people having an addiction to sugar, you need to know two things: it's real and it's dangerous. This goes beyond giving into a candy bar craving once in a while. People who are addicted to sugar eat large quantities of it every day. Sugar shows up in places you might not realize. It's recognized in junk foods like candy and cookies and ice cream. It can also be found in sodas and other sweetened beverages, breakfast cereals (even those that aren't targeted to children) and everyday staples such as bread, milk, yogurt and applesauce. It's possible you're addicted to sugar without even realizing it because the ingredient or ingredients like it - such as corn syrup - are added to a number of processed foods.

Why People Crave Sugar

There are a number of reasons that people crave sugar. One recent study out of Brazil linked stress to sugar cravings. Women who were experiencing high levels of stress were more likely to want sugar, and they were also more likely to have a larger waistline. It's also a learned habit. Once you start incorporating sugar into your daily diet, you begin to notice when you haven't had it in a while. That's how addictions work; the body needles the mind into thinking the substance is necessary. When your body grows accustomed to having a certain amount of sugar every day, those cravings will kick in until you satisfy the urge.

Hormonal changes in your body can also unleash a sugar craving. However, one of the most common reasons that people crave sugar is their body's response to insulin. If you have a poor diet that contains a lot of sugar and not enough vitamins and nutrients, your body has a hard time processing glucose, which is sugar broken down into its simplest form. The glucose can't get into your cells and it hangs out in your blood. This upsets the cells, which needs a certain amount of glucose to function, so they signal the brain to send down more sugar. This leads to sugar cravings and in some cases, diabetes.

The Addictive Properties of Sugar

The American Heart Association published a report with guidelines for sugar consumption. It advises men to eat fewer than 150 calories in sugar per day and women to keep their sugar calories at 100 daily. That report came after a California endocrinologist began studying the brain's response to sugar and compared it to the brain's response when it's addicted to cocaine. Neuroscientists have continued to study lab rats and confirm that sugar is just as addictive as drugs such as cocaine and heroin. The brain reacts similarly to the stimuli, whether it's a sugar filled cookie or a shot of cocaine.

There are also similarities in the processing of both drugs and sugar. Sugar in its natural form isn't so dangerous. Strawberries, for example, are loaded with natural sugars. However, they also have a lot of water and fiber which buffer the sugar before it can impact your healthy body. When the sugar is refined and processed, it becomes more potent and more dangerous. The same way that a poppy flower or a cocoa bean is harmless in its natural environment but dangerous and addictive when it's refined and turned into cocaine or heroin. It becomes habit forming and difficult to avoid.

Problems With Sugar Addiction

Sugar is a ready form of energy for the human body. However, consuming too much sugar may lead to tooth decay, weight gain, hypertension and diabetes. Sugar is the biggest culprit when it comes to tooth decay. Sugar provides fuel for the bacteria lurking in your mouth, resulting in increased acidity in your teeth and tooth decay.

When too much sugar is consumed, excess sugar is converted by the liver into fat for storage. Sugar triggers the release of insulin, which shuts down the fat burning process in the body and promotes the conversion of sugar into fat. Together these events cause weight gain, which if not controlled can lead to long-term complications such as hypertension and diabetes. Scientists are learning that sugar might be even more dangerous than salt when it comes to cardiovascular risks.

Too much sugar can also lead to liver problems and difficulties with your gastrointestinal tract. It tends to become a terrible cycle. The more sugar you eat, the more your body will crave it. Each day of too much sugar consumption makes it even more urgent for you to stop and moderate what you're eating; but at the same time each day makes it harder and harder for you to shut down the desire to eat it.

Sugar addiction is a learned habit. With modern food choices being what they are, children get addicted to sugar as soon as they are able to eat. It does not take them long to determine what tastes good, and if they are in a household where sugar is regularly consumed, their sugar addiction is locked into place even as their bodies are growing.

The addiction to sugar has become more widespread. People are constantly being lectured about their diets and their health and yet the trends of obesity, heart attacks, strokes and many kinds of cancer all point back to what people choose to eat and how they choose to live. The addiction to sugar is hard to break. It's not easy to change what you've learned. But if you want to live a long and healthy life - making that change is crucial.

Click the Link Below to Check out the Rest of "Sugar Detox" on Amazon

http://www.amazon.com/gp/product/B014I8OE3I?*Version*=1&*entries*=0

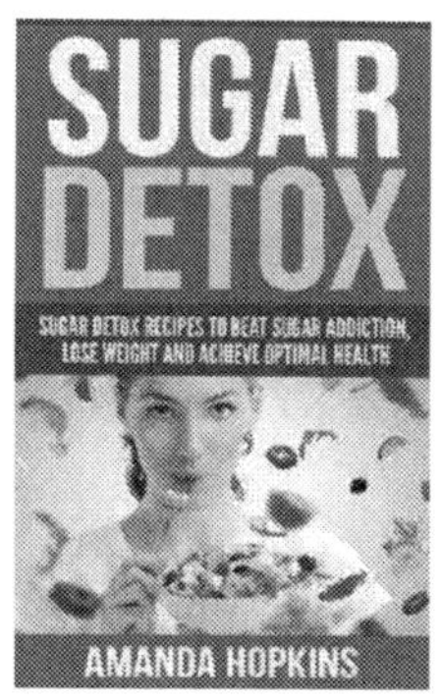

Check Out My Other Books

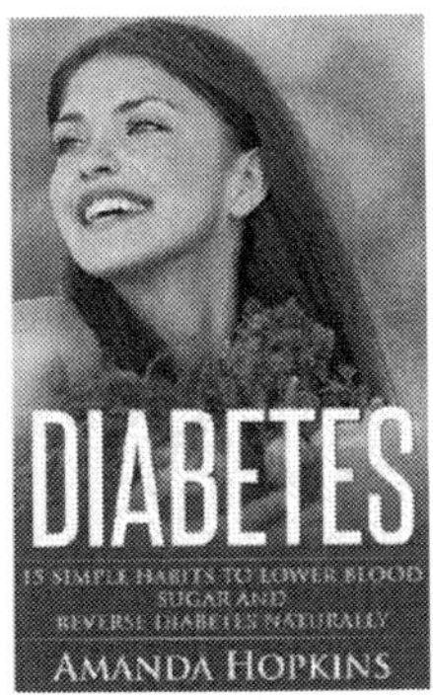

Diabetes: 15 Simple Habits to Lower Blood Sugar and Reverse Diabetes Naturally

http://www.amazon.com/gp/product/B00ZOBXQWE?*Version*=1&*entries*=0

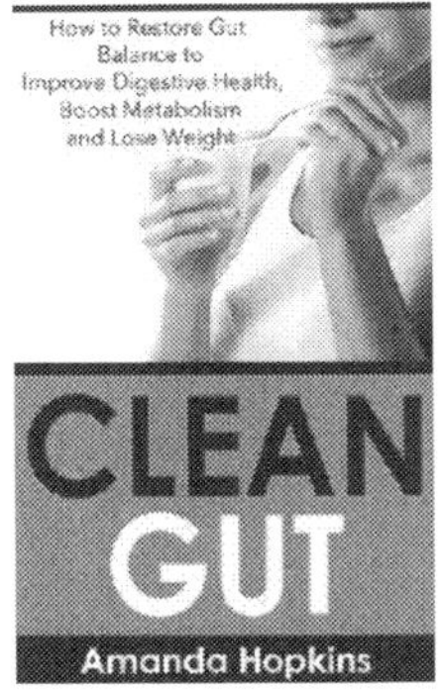

Clean Gut: How to Restore Gut Balance to Improve Digestive Health, Boost Metabolism and Lose Weight

http://www.amazon.com/gp/product/B0136XORHE?*Version*=1&*entries*=0

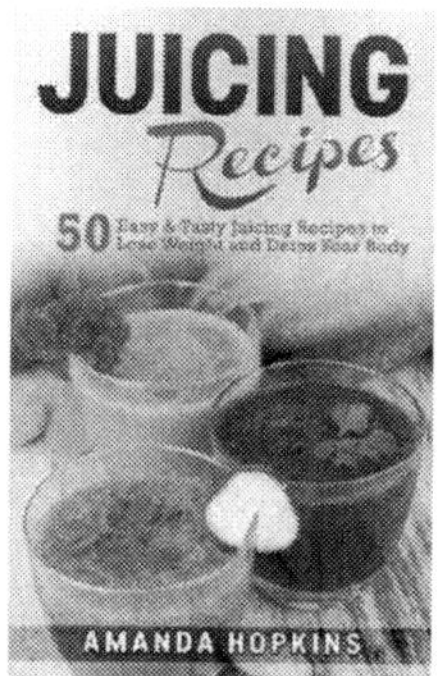

Juicing Recipes: 50 Easy & Tasty Juicing Recipes to Lose Weight and Detox Your Body

http://www.amazon.com/dp/B00UKHEP3Q

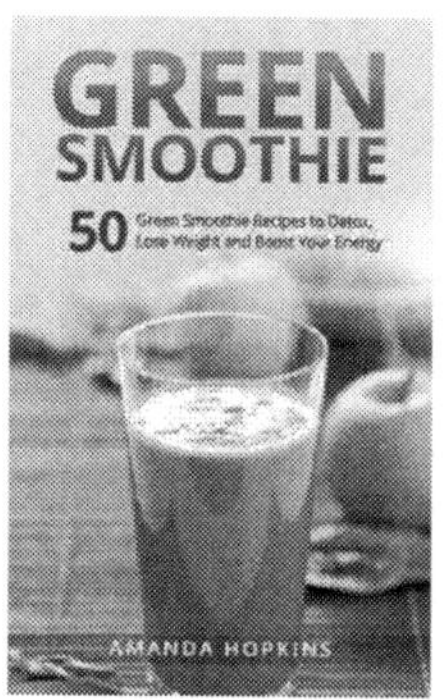

Green Smoothie: 50 Green Smoothie Recipes to Detox, Lose Weight and Boost Your Energy

http://www.amazon.com/dp/B00UMD97LS

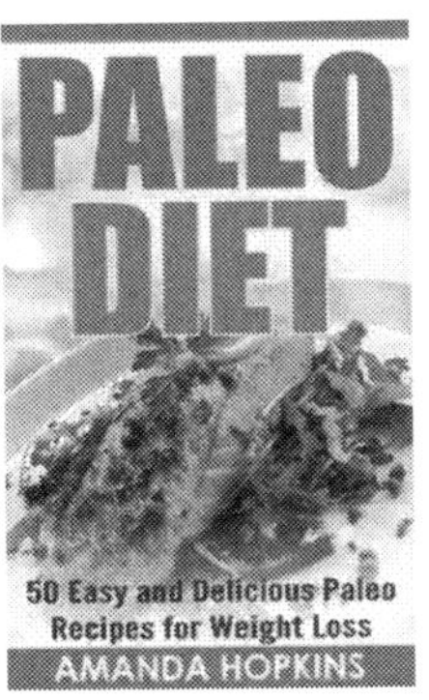

Paleo Diet: 50 Easy and Delicious Paleo Recipes for Weight Loss

http://www.amazon.com/dp/B00Y217JZM

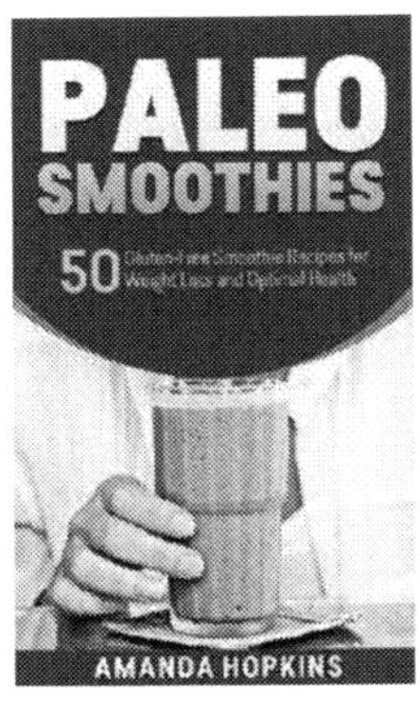

Paleo Smoothies: 50 Gluten-Free Smoothie Recipes for Weight Loss and Optimal Health

http://www.amazon.com/dp/B00X893X4U

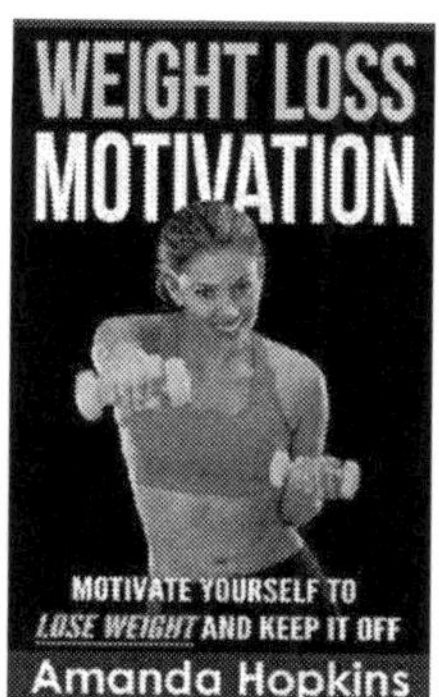

Weight Loss Motivation: Motivate Yourself to Lose Weight and Keep it Off

http://www.amazon.com/gp/product/B00S8PKOG4?*Version*=1&*entries*=0

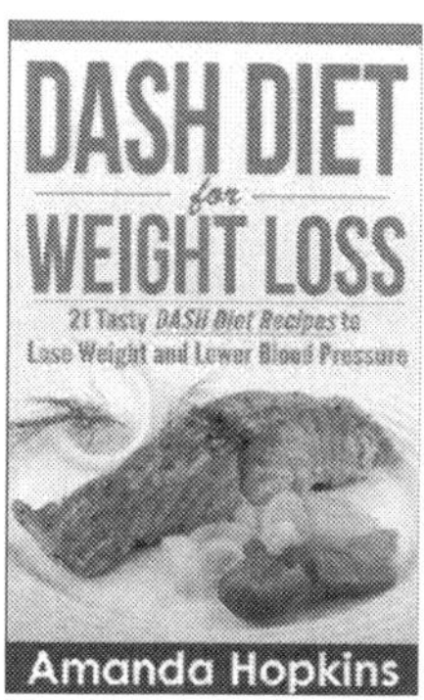

DASH Diet for Weight Loss: 21 Tasty DASH Diet Recipes to Lose Weight and Lower Blood Pressure

http://www.amazon.com/gp/product/B00SDMPIQI?*Version*=1&*entries*=0

Made in the USA
Middletown, DE
06 January 2020